Weight Loss

Making The Right Choice

Written by
Brenda Byrd

"The tragedy in life doesn't lie in not reaching your goal.
The tragedy lies in having no goal to reach."
Benjamin Mays

Table of Contents

Chapter 1:

Why Losing Weight Is Good

There is a great benefit acquired from losing weight. Though losing weight is not easy, the long term effects brought by it would probably be of help to anyone considering to shed those unwanted and unhealthy pounds.

The following are a few of the remarkable advantages from losing those excess weight.

Weight loss prevents high blood pressure, heart disease and stroke

That is a three in one benefit from losing weight. It is a fact that heart disease and stroke are one of the primary reasons for disability and death in both men and women in the US. People who are overweight have a higher risk to have high levels of cholesterol in their blood stream as well as triglycerides (also known as blood fat).

Angina, one type of heart disease, could cause chest pains as well as a decrease in the oxygen pumped to the heart.

Sudden death also occurs from heart disease and stroke, and usually this strikes with very little warning, signs and symptoms.

It is a fact that by decreasing your weight by a mere five to ten percent, this could positively decrease the chances of you having or developing heart disease or a stroke. Plus, how your heart functions would also improve as well as your blood pressure, cholesterol and triglyceride count will decrease.

Weight loss prevents type 2 diabetes

Diabetes puts in jeopardy one's life as well as how one leads his or her life because of the complications that result from having it. Both types of diabetes, type one and type two are linked with being overweight. To those who already have diabetes, regular exercise and losing weight could help in controlling your blood sugar levels as well as the medication you may be currently taking. Increase your physical activity. You could simply walk, jog or dance. It helps get those blood streams moving as well as lose those unnecessary pounds.

Weight loss helps reduce your risk for cancer

Being overweight is linked with a number of kinds of cancer. Specially for women, the common types of cancer that is associated with being overweight include cancer of the uterus, gallbladder, ovary, breast, and colon. This is not meant to scare you, this is only to keep you informed.

Men are at risk too from developing cancer if they are overweight. These include cancer of the colon, prostate and rectum. Extra weight, a diet high in fat and cholesterol should as much as possible be avoided.

Weight loss reduces sleep apnea

Or it could eliminate it all together. Sleep apnea is a condition wherein one could temporarily stop breathing for a brief period and then would continue to snore heavily. Sleep apnea could cause drowsiness or sleepiness during the day and – because of being overweight – could result in heart failure. Shedding those excess pounds could help in eliminating this problem.

Weight loss reduces the pain of osteoarthritis

When a person is overweight, the joints of his or her knees, hips and lower back have to exert double – if not triple – effort to carry him or her throughout his or her waking, walking and moving life. This could cause tension and stress on these joints. Weight loss decreases the load these joints carry thus decreasing – if not eliminating – the pain of one who has osteoarthritis.

Chapter 2:
Healthy Diet - A Guide To Weight Loss

Here are some weight loss diet tips that can be followed anywhere, everyday:

1. Make a delicious low fat mayonnaise by combining one teaspoon of Dijon mustard or satay sauce with a low fat yogurt.

2. Do not skip meals. Skipping meals slicks the body into slowing down the metabolism, attempting to conserve calories during a period where limited fats and fuel are available. Remember that eating increases the metabolism.

3. Stuff vegetables like capsicum and zucchini with flavored fillings or minced chicken, white meat or fish. These are healthy and contain low fat.

4. Take pita bread roll ups or wraps with salad fillings.

5. Eight hours after waking up, our metabolism slows down that is why 30 minutes of exercise before dinner will increase the metabolism for about two to three hours. This produces an increase in burned fat even hours after the work out is over.

6. Add alfalfa or mung beans to salad to get extra iron.

7. Good cooking and healthy eating begins with learning about nutrition and how to prepare healthy recipes.

8. Learn how to make the family favorite recipes and make sure that fats, salt, and sugar are cut out. Substitute non-fat yogurt for cream, stir-fry without oil and use herbs and spices instead of salt to taste.

9. Consult the doctor before beginning an exercise or weight loss program.

10. Slowly eat and chew each bite during meals as this would decrease one's appetite.

11. Complete three small meals and two snacks everyday instead of one or two huge meals.

12. Use chicken stock when stir-frying. This will cut down on hidden fat.

13. Buy non-toasted muesli instead of the toasted ones. A plate of toasted muesli contains more fat than a plate of bacon and eggs.

14. As much as possible do not remove the skins of fruits and vegetables since most of the nutrients are concentrated under the skin.

15. Warm water with just a squeeze of lemon juice before breakfast get the metabolism going for the day, this also help preventing constipation and is excellent for the skin.

16. One of the best sources of vegetable protein is from soya beans or tofu. All legumes provide some protein, so include lentils, lima beans etc into casseroles and soups.

17. Look for a weight loss "buddy," club, or support mates. This will motivate you to stay and enjoy your weight loss program.

18. Though it's hard at first, try not eating 3 hours or more before bedtime.

19. Make pasta a fast food choice - preparing a pasta meal or salad will only take 10-12 minutes.

20. Chilli helps to speed up metabolism - even the milder varieties.

21. Try making omelettes without adding the yolks! A dramatic decrease in fat.

22. Substitute baking soda, baking powder, MSG and soya sauce in cooking.

23. Remove fat by dropping ice cubes into the baking tray. Fat will stick to the ice cubes.

24. Drinking hot water instead of cold water in the morning can increase the speed of your metabolism and burn more calories.

25. Eat before you go food shopping and always prepare a shopping list. Only buy food which relates to your weekly menu plan and don't be tempted to buy goodies.

Make sure that the right discipline is still practiced to promote consistency on the diet plan. This will lead eventually to a healthy life-style and a more fruitful living without the extra fat and extra pounds on the side.

Chapter 3:
Weight Loss Tips

The good news is that there are a number of tips that you can use to help you successfully lose weight and hopefully achieve your weight loss goal.

When it comes to losing weight, the best thing that you can do is eat healthy. Eating healthy involves watching the foods that you eat, not necessarily how much food you eat. Of course, you may want to restrict the amount of foods that you eat, when on a diet, but it is more important to focus on the foods that you do eat. For instance, if you were to eat fruit instead of chips, you could have more fruit snacks with your meals than you would be able to if you were just to eat junk food.

Since eating healthy is an important component of losing weight, you may be wondering how you can go about doing so. One of the first things that you should do is find and familiarize yourself with healthy meals. You can do this by way of standard internet search or by buying a collection of healthy eating recipe books. To reduce the boredom often associated with healthy eating, especially if you are not use to it, it is important that you 'spice," up your foods and try to not eat the same meals over and over again each week.

In connection with healthy eating, regular exercise is also important to weight loss. If you are looking to lose weight, you should start an exercise plan for yourself.

Exercise is important as it burns off calories. When you burn calories, the amount of calories that your body absorbs decreases. This is, essentially, what makes it possible for you to lose weight.

If you haven't been exercising regularly in the past, it is important that you take it slow. Exercise is a great way to lose weight, but you do not want to overdo it, especially at first.

If you don't currently have an exercise plan or program in place, you may be wondering more about what you can do. One of the many ways that you can go about finding exercises or workouts to do is by buying a collection of fitness magazines. Many fitness magazines have detailed exercises outlined in them, often accompanied by pictures. You may also be able to find free instructional workout videos or exercise moves online. As a reminder, it is important to start out slow or at least start with exercises that would be easy for you to.

Eating healthy and regular exercise are both important components of losing weight, but there are additional tips that you can use to help you lose weight. One of those tips involves finding a workout partner or a workout buddy. This is a person who can exercise with you, whether your exercise involves visiting a local gym or just going for a walk at a local shopping center. Having a workout partner may help to keep you motivated and it may help to keep exercising and losing weight fun and exciting for you.

Another way that you can go about successfully achieving your weight loss goal is by 'spicing," up your exercises. As previously mentioned, you can use the internet or fitness magazines to find workouts for you to do at home.

To help reduce the boredom often associated with exercising you will want to change up your exercises, often on a daily basis. For instance, one day you may want to use a treadmill, the next day you may want to lift weights, and the next day you may want to do an exercise DVD, and so forth.

You should also consider making exercise and healthy eating logs or journals for yourself. These items can be used to track your progress. If you have a good week, like one where you completed all of your exercises, you may want to think about rewarding yourself. Your reward doesn't have to include food; it can be something as simple as a sticker or treating yourself to a movie.

Journals and logs have been known to help many individuals looking to lose weight and it may be able to do the same for you.

Chapter 4:
Visualization And Weight Loss - See The Pounds Drop Away!

The surprising fact is that many conditions can be improved by visualization and weight loss is one of them. It works like this: you keep a vision in your mind of how you want your body to look, and subconsciously you will begin acting in a way that will go in that direction. You become much more positive about your body, more a ccepting of your diet or fitness regime, and you will reach your weight goals more quickly and easily.

Effecting change through visualizing desired outcomes has become more and more acceptable in recent years. Psychologists do not understand exactly how it works but clearly the mind and body are not as separate as we often believe. It seems that if you truly want something it is more likely to happen - provided of course that it is some-thing that is possible, and within your control. Visualization helps us to truly want to lose weight by creating a clear and happy picture of our fitter bodies. Without this we can often put psychological traps in our own path.

Many people who are overweight believe they cannot lose weight. Sometimes you may say it out loud, or hear friends say it about themselves. For other people this belief stays in the subconscious. But it is sure that it influences our behavior. Someone who believes it is impossible for her to lose weight will be constantly battling her own negativity when she is trying to diet.

Her mind will be constantly telling her there is no point dieting, she cannot lose weight so she should just go ahead and eat everything she wants. Visualization is the strongest technique that we can use to overcome these negative thoughts and impulses.

If you are plagued by negativity either from your own mind or from the reactions of friends and family to your diet, go ahead and visualize yourself at your desired weight as often as you can. It works on the same level as all those negative voices and can annihilate their influence like nothing else can.

It is important to practice every day - morning and evening if you can. You just need to take a few minutes in a quiet place and keep an image in your mind of your body at its ideal weight. Some people can do this easily, others need some help. If you have a photograph of yourself at your ideal weight in the past, you may find it easier to look at that. Or use a photo from a magazine but cut off the person's face. You need to visualize your own body, but thinner.

You can also visualize from the inside. Close your eyes and let your awareness focus on a part of your body for example, your right thigh. Imagine it slowly becoming thinner in your mind's eye. Then move to the other thigh, and on through the body. It may help to start at the feet and move up towards the head, or vice versa.

As you go about your work or daily chores, think of your-self as already at your ideal weight. Create your own affirmations and repeat them often, always in the present tense ("I am glad to be flexible, fit and slim", not "I will ..."). Enjoy the feeling of having a positive self-image. Over time, this will help you to keep to your weight loss plan. You will find that fatty foods are less attractive and exercise is more enjoyable.

While your weight loss will of course be gradual, the wonderful thing about visualization is that it gives you a new body image right away. Use visualization and weight loss to make you happier right now, today!

Chapter 5:
Program Your Weight Loss In As Easy As A Week

The idea of the program is to be able for you to develop a consistent approach to weight loss as well as a healthy endurance when exercising. The program's objective is to get rid of the excesses in your body, the excess fat. Not the healthy and lean muscle tissues and body fluids.

The program first requires your focus and dedication, so therefore you need to be prepared in both mind and – of course – body. It is highly advised that you first visit your doctor for a check-up before embarking on any weight loss program.

It is important that when starting on any weight loss program, one should be positive enough to work for the results. Some people get impatient easily but long term effects are assured as long as one sticks to the weight loss plan at hand.

Stretch, stretch and stretch some more. Before actually doing those exercises and working out those muscles, a little stretching is needed in order to avoid any injury or soreness in your body.

It is also not advisable for anyone to try too hard. Everything should be done in moderation. Find the level of exercise and training that suits you. It should be enough for you to be comfortable in but not too convenient that it will not be much of a challenge. The first week

The first day of the program involves a long and steady walk in a little over twenty minutes. After the walk, follow it up with a good stretch. This takes so little of your time for the first day. In less than an hour you have taken that first step to a weight loss program that could work to your advantage.

By the second day, it is good to focus on an upper body workout. This maintains your strength to be able to go through the whole program for the week.

On the third day, a brisk walk or jog for ten minutes is in order. For beginners, a lower body workout should be done in the evening.

In the fourth day, a good rest is in order, as well as a good stretch. This lag time should be used wisely though to sort out any negatives in your mindset.

The fifth day starts with a good ten minute walk. Exercise the lower body in four sessions of workouts, follow this up with another ten minute walk, and another four sessions of lower body workout.

The sixth day should be spent on a low impact exercise such as swimming. To avoid boredom, do not be afraid to try something new. The last day of the week is a time to solicit the support of the people you care about. Spend time with them or get them to be with you in your long walk. Again, follow up your walk with a light upper body workout.

This is just the beginning though. If by this first week you are able to stick to the program, you have a great chance to further boost your weight loss and stay with the plan until you achieve your desired result.

Try as much as possible to be unlike the people who give up easily just because they could not see the result they want at the time they want – like this moment, today, now! Patience is a virtue.

The same way it took your body time to gain all that weight, think about it as the time your body will have to exert just to get rid of it.

Chapter 6:
Should You Join An Online Weight Loss Program?

Have you ever heard of an online weight loss program before? If this is your first time hearing about an online weight loss program, you may be wondering whether or not you should join one. If you are, you will want to continue reading on.

Perhaps, the biggest sign that you should think about joining an online weight loss program is if you are looking to lose weight. Whether you are interesting in improving your appearance, improving your health, or doing both, weight loss can be a stressful time.

Many weight loss programs assist you by having a daily food or exercise log for you to fill out. This has been known to motivate many online weight loss program members. Depending on the online weight loss program that you join, you should also get access to fun workouts and healthy recipes.

Another one of the many signs that you should think about joining an online weight loss program is if you regularly find yourself pressed on time. Whether you have a family to take care of, a demanding job, or both, you may find it difficult to eat healthy or maintain a regular exercise program. Joining an online weight loss program is a nice alternative to attending a local weight loss program, one that often requires you to meet for an hour or two a week.

Another one of the many signs that you should join an online weight loss program is if they are able to find an online weight loss program that is perfect for you. What is nice about online weight loss programs is that they come in a number of different formats.

For instance, it is possible to find "generalized," online weight loss programs, which are designed for all different individuals. On the other hand, there are themed weight loss programs, like ones that are designed for men, women, and senior citizens. Finding the perfect online weight loss program makes it well worth it for you to join one.

Speaking of finding the perfect online weight loss program, the best way to find one is to perform a standard internet search. When performing a standard internet search, you may want to search with phrases like "online weight loss programs," or "online weight loss plans." If you are looking for something specific, like an online weight loss program for women, you will want to incorporate that into your standard internet search. You can also ask those that you know for recommendations or find online discussions where online weight loss programs are being discussed.

When searching for an online weight loss program, you will likely come across multiple programs that may interest you.

When it comes to choosing an online weight loss program to join, it is advised that you take the features that you have access to, like online message board communication and healthy recipes, as well as costs into consideration. An online weight loss program that has more features or online resources for you may be worth paying a little bit more money for.

If you fit the above mentioned criteria, you may want to look into joining an online weight loss program. In fact, you may even find an online weight loss program that gives you a free trial period. This is the perfect opportunity to determine whether or not an online weight loss program is right for you.

Chapter 7:
Online Weight Loss Programs:
How They Work

Online weight loss programs are similar to many locally operated weight loss programs. Often times, the only difference is that you do not get to meet with group leaders or other members in person. If you are searching for a way to incorporate weight loss into your busy schedule, you are urged to examine online weight loss programs. These online weight loss programs are designed for all individuals, but they are perfect for those who regularly find themselves pressed for time.

When it comes to online weight loss programs, you will find that these online weight loss programs come in a number of different formats. For starters, it is possible to find free online weight loss programs; however, you will likely find that the best ones require the paying of a membership fee. Although each weight loss program is likely to vary, many have affordable monthly membership rates, some as low as five dollars a month. It is also possible to find weight loss programs that are designed for women, men, those over the age of fifty, and so forth.

If you have never joined an online weight loss program before, you may be wondering a little bit more about how they work. As previously stated, not all online weight loss programs are the same. With that in mind, however, you will find that many operate in similar matters. A few of the many member perks that you may get, when joining an online weight loss program, are outlined below.

One of the many perks or benefits to joining an online weight loss program is that you should get access to workout or exercise information. Many online weight loss programs will give you access to their website, which should have exercises and workouts outlined for you.

You should be able to get detailed directions for those exercises, pictures, and possibly even sample videos. Some more expensive online weight loss programs will give you access to customize workouts, ones which focus on the areas of your body that you would most like to improve.

Another member perk or feature that you should get access to with an online weight loss program is that of healthy recipes. Healthy eating is an important part of weight loss. That is why many online weight loss programs have a healthy eating section.
Not only may you get healthy food recipes, but you may also get money saving coupons, as well as cooking and food shopping tips.

As previously stated, often times the only difference between a locally operated weight loss program and an online program is the fact that you do not get to meet with the group leaders or other group members in person.

With online weight loss programs, you may not get in-person contact, but you may still be able to communicate. Many online weight loss programs have online message boards for their members to communicate with each other.

As a reminder, it is important to remember that not all online weight loss programs are the same. Despite the possibility of a variance, you should find that most online weight loss programs are more than worth your money, especially if you regularly find yourself pressed for time.

Chapter 8:
Paying For A Weight Loss Program Versus Developing Your Own

Whether you would like to improve your health, improve you appearance, or do both, you may be interested in finding a weight loss plan to use. When it comes to weight loss plans, you will find that you have a number of different options.

Two of your most common options include paying for a weight loss plan or developing your own.

If this is your first time attempting to 'seriously," lose weight, you may be wondering whether you should develop your own weight loss plan, also commonly referred to as a weight loss program, or pay for one. One of the best ways to determine which weight loss plan you should use is to examine the pros and cons of each. A few of the most influential advantages and disadvantages to developing your own weight loss plan, as well as paying for one are outlined below.

When it comes to paying for a weight loss plan or a weight loss program, you will find that you can do so locally or online.

If you choose to participate in a local weight loss program or plan, you will likely meet in a centralized location. Many times, you just get together every week or two. There are some weight loss programs where you can exercise onsite though. Should you choose to join an online weight loss program, you will likely have online meetings or discussions with trainers or other weight loss program members, either on a message board or through emails. You should also have access to healthy recipes and easy to do exercises.

One of the many advantages to paying for a weight loss program or a weight loss plan is that you are often given a professional plan. Many times, the individuals or trainers in charge of running these programs have training or firsthand experience with losing weight. This often eliminates trial and error, as many have already learned what works and what does not work with weight loss.

In all honestly, the only downside to paying to join a weight loss program or a weight loss plan is that you have to pay to do so. With that in mind, however, you should be able to find affordable weight loss programs and plans, both locally and online. Although it is not guaranteed, many people find the most affordable help in the form of online weight loss programs or online weight loss plans.

As for developing your own weight loss plan, there are a number of advantages to doing so. One of those advantages is that you can customize your weight loss plan and program to you. For example, if you were allergic to milk, you could work your allergy into your weight loss program, where as a paid weight loss plan or program may not do so.

You can also customize your workouts to yourself. This is great if you are obese and unable to follow many workout videos, which seem like they are designed for those who already in "perfect," shape.

Another one of the many advantages to developing your own weight loss plan to follow is that it is fun to do. You also have a number of tools at your fingertips. There are a number of websites and magazines that you can get weight loss information from; information that you can use to create your own weight loss plan to follow.

Some individuals have said that creating their own weight loss plan to follow makes them more excited about the process and more likely to see the plan all the way through.

The above mentioned factors are just a few of the many that you may want to take into consideration, when trying to determine whether you should develop your own weight loss program or join a paid weight loss program.

Many individuals have reported starting their own weight loss program and then later joining a paid one if they didn't get the results that they were hoping for.

Chapter 9:
Using The Internet To Develop Your Own Weight Loss Plan

Although you can pay to have a weight loss plan supplied to you or you can choose to join an existing weight loss program, you may find the cost of doing so a little bit difficult, especially if you are on a budget. That is why many choose to develop their own weight loss plans.

If this is your first time developing a weight loss plan for yourself, you may not necessarily know how you should proceed. What is nice about developing a weight loss plan for yourself is that you have freedom. With that in mind, you will still want to make sure that your weight loss plan is one that you can benefit from and one that you can lose weight while on. For that reason, you may want to think about turning to the internet, when looking to develop your own weight loss plan or weight loss program.

When it comes to using the internet to help you develop your own weight loss plan, there are a number of different ways that the internet can offer you assistance. For starters, a good part of a weight loss program involves eating healthy. For many individuals, eating healthy is something that is difficult to do, as they are unsure as to what they should cook or how they should cook it. There are a number of websites that you can find online, many of which are free to use, that give you access to healthy foods and recipes.

Many of these recipes are accompanied by pictures; therefore, you should be able to tell right away whether or not the food in question is something that you would eat.

Another part of losing weight involves exercise. For some individuals, taking a simple walk is enough to help them lose weight, but others must participate in more active exercise activities.

If you are one of those individuals, you can find a number of websites that outline exercises that you should be able to do. You will likely find a number of fitness websites that come with detailed pictures or videos, which outline each step of the workout in question.

You can also use the internet to order weight loss resources, like weight loss books or exercise equipment. One piece of exercise equipment that you may want to look into buy is that of an exercise video.

What is nice about using the internet to find an exercise video, which you can incorporate into your at-home weight loss program, is that you can not only buy videos online, but you can also find product reviews online.

Product reviews are a great way to determine if the exercise video you are interested in buying is really worth the money.

Once you have found a number of exercises that you would like to do or a number of healthy meals that you would like to make for yourself, you are advised to develop yourself a list, in writing or on the computer. This list can act as a schedule for yourself.

For instance, you could outline each workout that you would like to do on Monday's, as well as which meals you would like to eat on that same day. Having a detailed weight loss plan for each day of the week is likely to improve the chances of you following your own plan.

As you can see, the internet is a nice tool to have, when looking to create you own weight loss plan. For the best results, with finding what you need online, you may want to perform a standard internet search.

As a reminder, not everyone is able to develop their own at-home weight loss plans and follow them.

If you find that you are having a difficult time with staying on track, you may want to think about joining one of your local weight loss programs or even an online weight loss program.

Chapter 10:
Weight Loss Plan: The Goal To Go For

Since excess weight puts you at risk for many health problems, you may need to set some weight loss plans to help avoid those risks and prevent disease.

But what should be your long-term goal? And what short-term goals should you set to help you get there? You have a better chance of attaining your goals if you make sure that the weight loss plans that you will use are sensible and reasonable right at the beginning.

Here are some guidelines from the experts in choosing weight loss plans and goals.

1. Be realistic

Most people's long-term weight loss plans are more ambitious than they have to be.

For example, if you weigh 170 pounds and your long-term plan is to weigh 120, even if you have not weighed 120 since you were 16 and now you are 45, that is not a realistic weight loss goal.

Your body mass index or BMI is a good indicator of whether or not you need to shed of pounds. The ideal BMI range, according to the national Institutes of Health, is between 19 and 24.9. If your BMI is between 25 and 29.9, you are considered overweight. Any number above 30 is in the obesity range.

From this point of view, you will need a sensible weight loss plan that will correspond to the required BMI based on your height, because this is the primary factor that will affect your BMI.

2. Set appropriate objectives

Using a weight loss plan just for vanity's sake is psychologically less helpful than losing weight to improve health.

You have made a big step forward if you decide to undergo a weight loss plan that includes exercise and eating right so that you will feel better and have more energy to do something positive in your life.

3. Focus on doing, not losing

Rather than saying that you are going to lose a pound this week, say how much you are going to exercise this week. This would definitely make up of a sensible weight loss plan.

Keep in mind that your weight within a span of a week is not completely in your control, but your behavior is.

4. Build bit by bit

Short-term weight loss plans should not be "pie-in-the-sky." This means that when you have never exercised at all, your best weight loss plan for this week should be based on finding three different one-mile routes that you can walk next week.

5. Keep up the self-encouragement

An all-or-nothing attitude only sets you up to fail. Learn to evaluate your efforts fairly and objectively. If you fall short of some goals, just look ahead to next week. You do not need to have a perfect record.

After all, self-encouragement should definitely be a part of your weight loss plans. Otherwise, you will just fail in the end.

6. Use measurable measures

Saying that you are going to be more positive this week or that you are going to really get serious this week is not a goal that you can measure and should not be a part of your weight loss plan.

This is another reason why you should incorporate exercise on your weight loss plan and focus on it. You should be able to count up the minutes of exercise in order to be successful in your plan.

The bottom line is, people should make weight loss plans that will only remain as it is, just a plan. They have to put it into action by incorporating goals that will motivate them to succeed.

Chapter 11:
Weight Loss: Why Exercise Is Important

Are you interested in losing weight? If you are, you may be in the process of developing a weight loss plan for yourself. For many individuals, a weight loss plan is a guide that they can follow and one that may help to give them motivation. If this is your first time developing a weight loss plan for yourself, it is important that you place a focus on exercise, as exercise is important component of weight loss.

Although it is nice to hear that exercise is an important part of a weight loss plan, you may be wondering exactly why that is. For your body to lose weight, you must see a reduction in your calorie intake. The amount of calories that you need to reduce, in order to lose weight, will all depend on your current weight and your hopeful weight loss goal. Unfortunately, this is where many individuals automatically assume that they can't eat three meals a day and many actually just stop eating. This is not only dangerous to your health, but it can be deadly.

Instead of reducing your calorie intake by solely limiting the amount of foods that you eat, you can use exercise to your advantage. By exercising, you burn off calories. These are calories in which your body can use to help you lose weight. If you have a specific weight loss goal, like one that involves losing at least twenty pounds, you may want to focus on fun exercises or workouts, but also ones that burn the most calories. Adding exercise to your weight loss plan is a natural and a healthy way to lose weight.

Since it is important to incorporate to exercise into your weight loss plan, you may be wondering how you can go about doing so. In all honestly, there are an unlimited number of ways that you can go about using exercise to help you lose weight.

For starters, you can buy a collection, even just a small collection, of exercise equipment. Exercise equipment can include items such as exercise balls, weights, a treadmill, a stair climber, and so forth. Even if you have limited financial resources, you should be able to find a number of exercise equipment pieces that are within your budget.

Although you should be able to find a number of exercise equipment pieces, including instructional workout DVDs, for affordable prices, you may be looking to limit your weight loss plan investments.

If that is the case, you may want to take the time to examine your local gyms or fitness clubs. While some fitness clubs and gyms have relatively high membership fees, you can also find a number of them with affordable membership rates.

It is also important to mention that many fitness clubs and gyms are open accommodating hours, often making it easy to exercise before work, after work, or even during a lunch break of yours.

Despite the fact that exercise is often associated with exercise equipment, like a treadmill, that is not all that exercise is about. Exercise can also involve something simple like going for a walk or taking the stairs instead of the elevator at work. If you would prefer to exercise, for free, in your spare time, you may want to consider finding an exercise buddy.

This is a person who can workout with you, even if it just involves walking around your local shopping mall. Not only can you make a new friend or strengthen your relationship with one of your current friends, having an exercise buddy or an exercise partners often means that you are more likely to stick with your weight loss plan and achieve your weight loss goals.

As outlined above, it is extremely important that you incorporate exercise into your weight loss plan, especially if you are serious about losing weight and wish to do so in a healthy matter.

With multiple ways to go about incorporating exercise into your weight loss plan, there really isn't any excuse for not doing so.

Chapter 12:
What To Consider When Choosing An Exercise Video

If you are one of those individuals that wants to start your own plan, you may be interested in buying exercise videos. Exercise videos, also commonly referred to as workout videos, are a great addition to any weight loss program.

Although you may have bought workout videos before, have you even done so when seriously trying to lose weight? In the United States, a large number of individuals buy exercise videos just because. Just because exercise videos are a lot different than exercise videos that are a part of a weight loss plan. That is why you should shop for them differently.

When it comes to buying exercise videos for yourself, as a part of your weight loss program, there are number of important factors that you may want to take into consideration. These factors will not only make buying exercise videos for yourself easier, but they will also help to ensure that you choose the exercise video or videos that are best for you and your own personal needs.

A few of the many factors that you should take into consideration, when buying an exercise video are outlined below.

One of the many factors that you will want to take into consideration, when buying exercise videos as a part of your weight loss plan, is the type of exercises that you want to do. For instance, you often get to choose between traditional aerobic videos, yoga, Pilates, kickboxing, and so forth. To spice up your weight loss plan and to keep it fun and exciting, you may want to think about buying a collection of exercise videos, particularly a mixture of them.

Another one of the many factors that you will want to take into consideration, when buying an exercise video for your weight loss program, is difficulty. What you need to remember is that many workout videos come in sessions. For instance, it is possible to find kickboxing videos that are designed for beginners, those at the intermediate level, as well as those at an advanced level. You want to make sure that you choose the right video for yourself. If you are not careful, you may end up with an advanced workout video that you cannot even use, as you are unable to keep up with the instructor.

Cost is another factor that you may want to take into consideration, when buying workout videos or exercise videos for yourself. In your search for exercise videos, you will find that they are sold for a wide range of prices. Some are affordable, others are a little bit more costly, and many are downright expensive.

Of course, the expensive workout videos may be worth the cost, but you never really know until you order them. One way to help make sure that you are spending your money wisely is to search for exercise video reviews online. This can often be done with a standard internet search.

The above mentioned factors are just a few of the many that you may want to take into consideration, when buying exercise videos to incorporate into your at-home weight loss program. Most times, you will find that any exercise video is better than no video at all, but taking the time to find the perfect one will likely make your weight loss program much more enjoyable.

Chapter 13:
Understanding Natural Weight Loss

The experts in weight loss and diet programs are continuously struggling to give weight loss clients the best possible answer to their weight problems. And the latest trend introduced is natural weight loss. So what is this natural weight loss thing?

Natural Weight Loss Explained

Since the procedures are natural, weight loss using this procedure is considered healthy and will really make you feel satisfied. Unlike the fad diets and "almost magic" diet programs and medications available today, natural weight loss will teach you how to shed those extra pounds in a proper manner.

This weight loss means will tell you the opposite of what those unreliable diet programs tell you; that you will lose weight if you are going to religiously follow a long term but healthy weight loss plan.

Now, don't you think it is much easier to believe in a weight loss procedure which does not promise making you sexy and fit overnight? But, what can you really do to lose weight naturally?

Here are some tips;

• Know what to eat

It is important that you know whether a certain food on your menu can be a potential harm to your weight loss scheme. Learn how to be critical on what you eat. Avoid too much fried and salty foods.

• Read about natural weight loss

There are lots of published, both online and prints, about natural weight loss. It would help you so much to read on some of these articles. You can read books or magazines with expert's column about natural weight loss. Online natural weight loss sites are also available on the net as your reference.

• Participate on online forums

Yes, there are online communities and forums on the Internet where members talk about natural weight loss, its benefits and the different resources which you can find to shed that unwanted fat naturally.

• Visit websites

There are different natural weight loss websites and you can visit any of them so you can get guides about losing weight. You'd be able to get tips and information about natural weight loss programs and pills on such sites.

• Don't believe in magic

When it comes to losing weight, there is no such thing as magic. Patience and perseverance are what you need.

Really, there are lots of ways for you to be fit the natural way. You just have to know the different resources that you have. And after some time, you will feel the difference between the commercial diet solutions and the natural way. It is because eventually, you will become perfectly fit while staying healthy. Yes, healthy because you are not restricting yourself with what you eat.

With natural weight loss, you don't deprive yourself. You just learn what are the right amount and the right time to eat them. And you know what? Permanent fitness is the promise of losing weight naturally. That's right; you don't have to worry about gaining weight again.

Chapter 14:
The "quick Weight Loss Diet"
Trend Disadvantage

If you wear a size 14 and you blow a bundle on designer size 8 dresses as motivation, you will probably end up feeling guilty, frustrated, and angry if you are not slinking around in it a month later.

In reality, you will do much better setting smaller, achievable targets for yourself. If you must try the new-clothes strategy, go down a size at a time, and do not buy anything you have to take out a second mortgage to pay for.

Because, if you continue to remorse on losing weight fast, you will end up incorporating fad diets or those that offer quick weight loss.

For most people who are not aware of this fact, there are no such things as quick weight loss diets and there is no nippy weight loss for people who want to be slimmer than what their body can provide.

The problem with most people is that they tend to opt for nippy fixes wherein fact these things are not effective at all.

What Does Not Work

Today, there are plenty of weight-loss strategies that are guaranteed to backfire. This is because these nippy fixes instilled on certain diet plans are, in reality, not efficient because it does not employ the right principle and the right attitude in losing weight.

These quick weight loss diet plans are known as fad diets because that is exactly what they are, just a fad. In time, when fashion is over and popularity wanes down, people will realize that the diet they have depended on is not reliable at all.

To know more about these fad diets that are selling like hotcakes in the market today, here is a list of some telltale signs that would tell you not to try it even once.

Here they are:

1. Skipping meals

Does your diet plan require you to skip meals? If it does, then, it is a fad diet.

Abstain from food completely is not a healthy habit. It may even cause some serious complications or problems especially for people who are sick with diabetes.

Skipping meals will only cause a hypoglycemia, or the condition wherein your blood sugar is really low, and will probably only be effective in making you eat twice as much at the next meal.

2. Dieting without exercise, or vice versa

Exercise is crucial to the human body. It is important in the proper blood circulation and other activities of the human body system. Therefore, diet plans that do not require you to exercise are nuisances. People are born to move.

But then again, exercise alone is not sufficient. Hence, it would be better if diet and exercise will go hand-in-hand.

3. Continuous dawdling

There is no better time to start losing weight. If you want to really lose those excess fats, you have to lose weight now.

Delaying tactics will not get you anywhere and will only make the problem worse. So, if your diet plan suggests a certain time frame for you start losing weight, chances are, you are following the trend of fad diets.

Boiled down, it is best to rely more on the way you feel than the tale of the tape. This means that if the weighing scale tells you that you are losing weight even if it is slower than you would like, but you are feeling energetic and positive about your weight-loss efforts, then, you are just doing fine.

As mentioned and is worth mentioning all over again, weight loss is not a quick process.

Chapter 15:
The Dangers Of Rapid Weight Loss

Rapid weight loss, also commonly referred to as quick weight loss or fast weight loss, involves losing weight in a short period of time, often anywhere from two to seven days.

Each year, in the United States, hundreds of thousands of Americans are interested in rapidly losing weight. Many people wish to lose weight before an important event, like an upcoming vacation or a wedding.

While it is defiantly possible to understand how you can want to lose weight quickly, namely as fast as possible, you need to proceed with caution. Although it is possible to lose weight, at least a little bit of it, in a relatively quick period of time, you should know that there are dangers associated with doing so.

One of the many dangers of rapid weight loss is some of the many measures that some people take. For instance, it is common to hear of individuals who have decided not to eat, while trying to achieve a rapid weight loss.

Going without food, for even a short period of time, can be dangerous to your health. A better alternative is to cut back on the food that you do eat or to just make sure that it is healthy foods in which you are eating. By limiting your calories, you should be able to achieve at least a small weight loss in the time that you were looking to. It is just very important that you do eat.

In addition to eating healthy, another component of weight loss is exercise. Unfortunately, many individuals do not realize that it can take up to one week to notice the signs of exercise. With that in mind, the more weight you need to lose, the sooner it is that you may start seeing results.

While exercise is a major component of losing weight, it is important that you do not overdo it, especially if you haven't had a regular exercise plan. Running on the tread-mill for three hours, instead of thirty minutes, may help re-duce your calorie intake, but, at the same time, it may also land you in the hospital.

Another problem that is often associated with rapid weight loss is the taking of medications or other weight loss products. The good news is that many of these products do work and some are even safe, but you may not be able to tell what you are getting.

If you are interested in using a weight loss product, like a diet pill or a cleanse, to help you lose weight, it is important that you do the proper amount of research first.

This research may involve checking product reviews, to see if the product is effective, or speaking with a health-care professional.

As you can see, it is important that you proceed with caution when trying to achieve rapid weight loss. Although unexpected events or appearances do pop up, most individuals have at least a months worth of notice before attending a large event, like a wedding or even a vacation.

As soon as you know about your upcoming event, you are advised to start trying to lose weight then, if you are interested in doing so. Rapid weight loss can be dangerous; therefore, you shouldn't rely on it if possible.

Chapter 16:
What Is In A Weight Loss Diet Pill?

With all the strenuous activities and sweat-generating regimens that most weight loss programs have, more and more people are enticed to opt for a better alternative, without the trouble of exerting too much effort.

With the advent of diet pills that promote weight loss, people go mad over the appealing advertisements of most manufacturers claiming that their product can easily 'melt away" those fats and cellulite.

With these pills dominating the market today, who needs to tone those abs and biceps and do some dieting if there is an easier way to lose weight?

With an estimated 60% of the American population that are now considered as obese, these "wonder" drugs are definitely reaping millions of dollars in the United States alone.

Now, the questions are: is there any truth regarding the manufacturers" claims that these diet pills can ultimately promote weight loss? Are they really effective in helping people lose weight? And if that is the case, do these pills also help those people maintain their ideal weight and curb any fat accumulation in the body?

In reality, there are diet pills that can really make a person shed off those extra pounds. These diet pills contain certain substances that were already clinically and scientifically proven to be very effective.

These diet pills are effective in increasing the metabolism of the body, thereby, initiating weight loss. Plus, these diet pills contain certain substances that suppress one's appetite.

However, with so many diet pills saturating the market today, trying to find the best and most effective diet pill can be very tedious. Chances are, you may end up choosing the wrong diet pill when your energy to find diet pills wanes down.

Actually, there are only five factors to consider when choosing diet pills that are effective at the same time safe to use. Here is a list of the factors that you need to consider in order to come up with a diet pill that is right and appropriate.

1. The metabolism-boosting ability

In choosing diet pills that will effectively promote weight loss, it is best to look for pills that have the ingredients that will enhance your body's metabolism, or the ability of the body to burn excess fats.

Choose those diet pills that contain alpha lipoic acid, green tea extracts, and "L-Canitine" because these ingredients had been clinically proven to be effective in promoting weight loss through increased metabolic rate.

2. The appetite suppressants

Find diet pills that effectively suppress your appetite. It does not necessarily mean that you will skip meals but you will not just feel hungry every now and then. This is because obesity usually happens to people who are fond of in-between meals, which actually initiates excessive calorie intake.

3. The calorie stopper

Because obesity is usually due to excess intake of calories in the body, which is more than the recommended amount, it is best to choose diet pills that have the special ingredients that will curb the entry of calories into the body.

These substances are known as "phaseolus vulgaris." This is known to create an enzyme that will efficiently control any excess calories in the body. The enzyme responsible for this wonderful job is known as "alpha-amylase."

4. The metabolic enhancers

It is best to choose diet pills that have the so-called "lipotropic elements" that are effective in eliminating fats from the body. It functions like a sweeper that effectively sweeps excess fats outside the body.

These lipotropic elements are found in vitamin C, chitosan, alpha lipoic acid, and green tea extracts.

5. The water-retention breaker

Effective diet pills are those that contain diuretics. These are elements that avert the retention of water in the body during the weight loss regimen.

All of these factors are, indeed, clinically proven and effective in losing weight. Though, it must be kept in mind that diet pills alone are not sufficient to provide optimum weight loss. Hence, it is still important to do some exercises.

Therefore, with exercise and the right diet pills, you are definitely on your way to a healthier, slimmer you.

Chapter 17:

Nutrition Notes On Weight Loss Supplements

More and more spend hundred and even thousands of dollars yearly on weight loss supplements in the hope of speeding up their metabolism. The main desire is to be attractive and accepted but it is becoming a more difficult goal to achieve.

The fitness industry is booming but still a lot of people are unable to cut those fat in spite of all the exercise and diet efforts. In America, more than sixty per cent of adults are overweight and thirty per cent are considered obese.

This is because:

1, a lot of weight loss products promises unrealistic goals;

2, dietary supplement manufacturers rely on the overweight person's failure to survive; and three, the information about the supplements in the market are just written by themselves just to make a sell.

Although the Food and Drug Administration has successfully banned illegal marketers, some products are still available. Consumers can be deceived of the labels which claims caffeine or ephedra fee not knowing that these supplements composes of other ingredients that may pose the same health risks. These include heart and digestive problems, headaches, insomnia, and even psychological side effects.

Other supplement manufacturers say that their products contains EGCG which is a phytochemical ingredient found in green tea. This so-called component claims to speed up metabolism but in reality poses to reduce the risk of cancer.

Some studies denote that it could slightly increase the potential to burn calories and now can be found in many weight loss supplements. It has good points on the other hand since the body might conform to EGCG after a period of time. Eve the weight loss benefit could sum up to 60 to 70 calories a day. This helps prevent excessive weight gain.

A few other significant effects of weight loss supplements is that it may contain ingredients that makers claim will prevent the absorption of carbohydrates. One good example is Chitosan, which appears most promising, which in fact shows no positive result in fat absorption.

It could even take up to seven months for men to lose just a pound of body fat and for women, there is no fat loss at all. Thyroid supplements act as thyroid replacements help regulate and optimize the thyroid at a higher level. This they say makes the body feel like a couch potato and won't perform the job it has to.

Since the number one reason why people eat is because they feel hungry, there is another type of ingredient that manufacturers made which increases the feeling of being full and decreases appetite, Guar Gum. However, recent studies show that it has no meaningful benefit at all to weight loss. It is ironic that manufacturers mix Psyllium that has the reputation of reducing eating and aiding weight loss for initial studies so far do not support this claim although it helps control blood cholesterol and sugar.

One of the latest innovations in the fat loss industry is by way of skin absorption. There's a Cutting Gel, which is an epidril product by far the best selling in fat loss creams technology. Rub it where you want the fats cut. For now, it will seem safer to advise the age old remedies to excess-ive weight gain and that is to invest on walking shoes instead of diet supplements, go to the park and do brisk walking, go to the gym, and have a well balanced diet in-stead.

Chapter 18:
Tablets To Help In Weight Loss

Recent studies have shown that more people are getting overweight every year. This happens not only to adults but even to kids who have just started in school.

There are many factors that have contributed to this such as the rise in the number of fast foods joints that contain a lot of saturated fat in the meals, the use of refined sugar in sodas and other processed foods, eating food with less fiber, genetics, overeating and as people age slow metabolism.

Since losing weight takes time and most people can't wait to get rid of it, these people have decided to take the fastest way out which is through the use of weight loss tablets.

In the 1950's until the late 90's, doctors prescribed drugs for weight loss. The drug works by increasing the serotonin levels in the brain that makes the brain believe that the stomach is already full and thus, increases the person's metabolic rate.

It was only after scientists discovered that these drugs had side effects and were related to cause heart valve disease that these were taken off the shelves.

Later on, modifications have been made and new drugs were developed and prescribed by doctors and many of which are still waiting for FDA approval.

The idea that a simple drug can change everything without the need to change ones diet or sacrificing anything is very tempting since people have seen friends and family members use it and have shown tremendous improvement.

This has made a lot of people spend millions of dollars every year to also experience this miracle and has given drug companies a lot of money making the drug and selling it.

Diet pills can be purchased either over-the-counter or prescribed by a doctor. Even with the advances in medical technology, these drugs still pose a health risk to the public. Problems in patients can be unpleasant such as diarrhea and vomiting, harmful such as tightness in the chest and in the urinary tract and fatal such as a heart attack or a stroke.

An overdose in using weight loss tablets can cause tremors, confusion, hallucinations, shallow breathing, renal failure, heart attack and convulsions.

The side effects vary depending on the lifestyle and health of the person and can be minimized as long as one consults the doctor and follows the prescribed dosage when using it.

Should one decide to stop using the drugs, studies have shown that a person will experience withdrawal symptoms and side effects. These include noticeable mood swings, hyper-activity, and pain in the stomach, insomnia and nightmares, severe irritability, extreme fatigue, depression, nausea, vomiting and trembling.

A lot of clinical tests will show that the taking this weight loss tablets really work. But this can only work if it is done with a low calorie diet and an exercise plan.

A person can jog every morning or sign up and workout in a gym. Just like taking any medicine, one should first consult the doctor before undergoing any form of exercise.

The best exercise plan should have cardiovascular and weight trainingexercises.
This helps burn calories and increase the muscle to fat

ratio that will increase ones metabolism and lose weight.

It is up to the person already to stick to the program to see that it works.

Chapter 19:
Weight Loss Products: How To Spot A Scam

Are you looking to lose weight? If you are, there is a good chance that you will start your own weight loss program. When many individuals start their own weight loss programs, they do so with the help of a number of weight loss products, like diet pills or exercise equipment. If you are interested in buying these types of weight loss products, you need to always be on the lookout of scams, as they do exist.

When it comes to weight loss products, like exercise equipment and diet pills, many people automatically wonder how they can tell if they are being scammed. Unfortunately, you often cannot tell by reading an advertisement in a magazine or online or by watching a television infomercial or even by looking at the weight loss product in question. The best way to determine if the weight loss product you are interested in buying is really worth your money is to do research first.

When it comes to researching weight loss products, there are a number of different ways that you can go about determining if the product or products you want to buy are worth the cost. One of the easiest ways to go about doing so is by visiting the online websites of retailers that allow their customers or the general public to rate or review their products. Many consumers like to alert others to a product that is a waste of money or even alert others to a product that is well worth the cost. If you are able to find weight loss product reviews, you are advised to read them.

When reading weight loss product reviews, like product reviews for diet pills or exercise equipment, it is important to remember that no product is perfect. Even the best products, like the ones that come highly rated and recommended, will have a few bad reviews.

What you need to be cautious of is any weight loss product that has more bad reviews than it does good reviews. This is a surefire sign that the weight loss product in question may not be worth your money.

You can also find product reviews or just specific weight loss products being discussed by performing a standard internet search. When performing a standard internet search, you will want your search phrase to be the name of the weight loss product in question.

Your standard internet search may lead you to online message boards where weight loss and other health issues are being discussed. These types of websites and message boards are a great way to also learn about weight loss products that you may not have otherwise came across.

Another way that you can determine if you are being 'scammed," by a weight loss product, is by examining the online website of the product distributor or manufacturer.

When you buy a diet pill or another weight loss supplement, you should be provided with as much information as possible. Be cautious of any product whose website only claims to help you lose weight, but doesn't explain how it is done. The same can be said for exercise equipment.

Another great way that you can determine if the weight loss products you are interested in buying are worth the money is by speaking with your doctor. Often times, you don't even have to schedule a visit; a telephone call should get you the answers that you were looking for.

Most doctors can let you know if a weight loss pill or supplement that you are interested in buying is worth the money. If they can't tell you about the specific product in question, there is a good chance that they can at least review the ingredients with you. For exercise equipment, your physician may also be able to provide you with advice.

Of course, if you have the money to spend on weight loss products, you may be interested in going ahead and buying the product or products in question anyways.

That is fine to do, but you also need to remember that many weight loss products, especially the ones featured on television infomercials are priced relatively high.

Chapter 20:
Weight Loss Exercise Products You May Want To Buy

Are you interested in losing weight and improving your appearance? If you are, you should know the importance of exercise.   Exercise burns off calories, which reduces your calorie intake, which, in turn, makes it possible for you to lose weight.

If this is the first time that you have decided to seriously try to lose weight, you may be looking to buy exercise equipment for yourself. If you are, you will want to continue reading on. Below, a few popular pieces of exercise equipment that you may look into buying are outlined.

One piece of exercise equipment that you may want to look into buying is that of a treadmill. Treadmills are, per-haps, the most well-known piece of exercise equipment available. What is nice about treadmills is that they come in a number of different styles.

For instance, you can find treadmills that are powdered by electricity and then treadmills that are powdered by your own walking. This is nice as it often results in treadmills being available for a wide range of prices. Whether you have one hundred dollars to spend on a treadmill or one thousand dollars, you should be able to find a treadmill for your home weight loss plan.

Another piece of exercise equipment that you may want to look into buying, for your at-home weight loss plan, is that of an elliptical machine. Elliptical machines are nice, as they often combine multiple exercises. More advanced elliptical machines, also commonly referred to as deluxe elliptical machines, often given you an upper body workout and a lower body workout as well. Elliptical machines are often referred to as combination stair climbers and ski machines.

An exercise bike is another popular piece of exercise equipment that you may want to think about buying for your at-home weight loss program. Like an elliptical machine, there are many exercise bikes that give you an upper body and a lower body workout.

These are points to take into consideration, should you decide to buy an exercise bike for yourself. Like tread-mills, exercise bikes come in a number of different formats and styles; therefore, they are sold for a wide range of prices.

One piece of exercise equipment that you may not necessarily think about buying, but one that you should examine is that of a trampoline. When it comes to trampolines, you will find that they come in a number of different formats. For instance, it is possible to find larger size trampolines, ones that are ideal for backyards and often associated with recreational play. While these trampolines can also be used for exercise, there are smaller, mini trampolines that are designed for exercises, as well as indoor use. These types of trampolines are often fun, exciting, and affordable.

The above mentioned pieces of exercise equipment are ones that are often larger in size and occasionally more expensive. If you are looking for more affordable pieces of exercise equipment or more compact pieces, you still have an unlimited number of products to choose from.

For instance, there are yoga and Pilates items that are often affordable and small in size. Exercise balls and resistance bands are popular items that you may want to take the time to examine. There are also weight sets that you can buy or you can buy a few individuals weights to use at home. When it comes to exercising at home, your options are, literally, unlimited.

When it comes to buying exercise equipment for yourself, you will find that you have a number of different options. You can shop locally or online. Exercise equipment is sold at sports stores, as well as traditional department stores.

If you are on a budget, you may want to look into buying used exercise equipment. Used exercise equipment can often be found on online auction websites, in thrift stores, and at yard sales.

As outlined above, there are a number of different exercise equipment pieces that you can use to help you lose weight at home. Whether you choose to buy some of the pieces outlined above or something else, you are sure to have a fun and exciting time working to achieve your weight loss goal.

Chapter 21:
Natural Weight Loss Remedies - Thermocerin

Don't think that changing your diet and exercising is going to really cut it? Turns out you're not alone. Literally thousands of people are trying to find natural weight loss remedies to trim down.

Being over weight, now regarded by many as a medical condition, is actually something YOU can cure. With a little help, you may be able to kick start your weight loss program with the natural weight loss remedy Thermocerin.

Going into this you already likely know there is no such thing as a miracle solution. Hard work is the key, after all you likely did not put the weight on over night, so it isn't going to come off over night either. But, there's actually more to it - a reason your body objects to losing weight - biochemical and biological reasons. In short form, your fat cells are working against you. The first thing you do when you go on a diet is reduce your caloric intake. That makes your body panic, and it starts thinking you're starving it.
So instead of going WITH the program, they store the fat for later, just in case. How annoying. This reaction is caused by fat receptors. They want to go into hoard

mode. So you need to find a way to turn the fat receptors off and release fat into your bloodstream and burn it. The product Thermocerin claims that it teaches your body thermogenesis - tells your fat cells to shut up and get on the same page towards weight loss, not retention.

Thermogenesis means your body produces heat or energy through a chemical reaction. The more energy produced, the higher your metabolic rate and the more fat gets burned. So, if your metabolism is higher due to more energy being generated you are benefiting from the thermogenic effect - the increased burn off of calories and fat. It also goes hunting to find stored fat and burns it out was well.

So what's in Thermocerin? The short answer is polyphen-ols(plant chemicals creating pigment) from green and white tea plants plus Capsaicin (active component in chili peppers) and Yohimbe.(antioxidant properties).
Will it work? Anecdotal evidence suggests it will, but with any product that has a combination of herbs in it, natural or not, you should make certain to do your research first. This is even more important if you happen to have an allergy to herbs. So make sure you read the fine print and look things up on the Internet.

Chapter 22:
Fad Diets: Why Are They Bad?

It is not surprising that many people wonder why fad diets are bad when they seem to get results. You will find many sites on the internet claiming significant weight loss in just a few days. That type of weight loss is always temporary.

It is usually 90% water which will be put straight back on as soon as your body rehydrates, which it must do if you are not going to suffer severe health problems or die.

Other fad diets are not so obviously crash diets with outrageous claims but they are over hyped diet plans that tend to be fashionable for a while and usually make a lot of money for the inventor in associated product sales.

In the best cases these are good nutrition plans which will help you lose weight, but which you could probably have gotten for free from your doctor. In the worst cases they will prove so difficult to follow that you will give up after a week.

The bad of fad diets

1. Diets that promise quick and easy weight loss are usually based on eating more of one food type and none of another. These do not give the benefits that you would get from a balanced diet. They may suggest you take supplements but many supplements are not absorbed by the body unless they are taken along with the foods that the diet has banned. After a few weeks, if you stick to it that long, you may begin to develop nutritional deficiencies.

2. Fad diets are often boring and over restrictive. After the novelty of the first day or two, you will not enjoy your meals. You will then start to crave food constantly and will break the diet. You may even feel guilty, thinking it is your fault that you did not lose weight.

3. Most fad diets do not follow recommendations of the American Heart Association and similar bodies for fat levels in the diet. Often the diet will recommend high fat foods and low carbs which if taken long term, could result in heart disease.

The promoters may tell you that the diet is only intended to be followed for a short time. But you probably will not reach your goal weight in that time, and then what? You either continue with a plan that is not good for your health, or stop and probably gain back what you lost.

4. Many fad diets do not help you to incorporate enough servings of fruits and vegetables in your weight loss program, or give you the variety of foods that your body needs.

5. Quick weight loss diets are just a temporary solution and do not help you to make permanent changes to your eating habits. Permanent changes are the only way to remain at your target weight once you reach it. Fad diets encourage yo-yo diet-binge cycles of fast weight loss and equally fast weight gain. This is worse for your health and your self esteem than if you had stayed overweight all the time.

Whatever the publicity materials may say, these diets will not help you in the long term. The best way to sustain weight loss is to eat a varied and healthy diet, do not overeat, exercise regularly and avoid fad diets.

Chapter 23:
Exercise Is The Best Way To Lose Weight

There are a lot of people who are overweight. This did not happen overnight so those who think this can disappear in a flash should think again.

There are many ways that the person can use to get rid of those excess pounds. Although science has developed diet pills and some have developed diet programs, the best way to lose weight is still through exercise.

Exercise is the best because it builds the person's endurance. As this develops, it also increases ones metabolism prompting one to burn more calories than before which results in weight loss.

Studies show that there are no known side effects when one decides to exercise. The worse that can happen to a person is straining a muscle for failing to stretch or by not giving the body enough time to recuperate before engaging in another session.

Teens don't have to spend much in order to lose weight. This is because there are some exercises that can be done at home. For instance, after stretching, the person can go for a walking or jogging early in the morning thus burning a few calories. Afterwards, the teen can do some push ups and sit ups to work on the upper body and the abs.

The other way that will cost a little will be by enrolling in a gym. Here, a fitness trainer can help the individual lose weight by coming up with a program that involves cardio-vascular and aerobic activity.

Warm up will be running for a few miles on the treadmill followed by some weight training using the various machines.

Teens who find it difficult to hire a trainer can make a workout after being taught how to use the equipment while those who have fun with many people around can join one of the classes being offered at the gym.

Some of the more popular group classes are aerobics, tae bo, Pilates and yoga. The person should just check what time the classes are held since this may be scheduled at different times of the day.

Those who are shy about being with other people but would still like to participate in a class can get the DVD version instead.

There are a lot of these being sold in the video store or online which is just like being there and attending the real session.

One of the most important things to remember while exercising is to drink lots of water. People who fail to do this may suffer from heatstroke or dehydration which is also not good for someone who wants to lose weight.

Before engaging in any exercise, it is advisable to see a doctor. The mind may feel like it can do anything but if the body may say differently. The teen should just do things gradually at first and then pick up the pace with other exercises as time progresses.

Engaging in a sport is another form of exercise. Running down the court in a game of basketball or football may not seem like much but it still increases one's heart rate and burns those calories.

These examples just show that there are many ways how a teen can lose weight. There are people out there who sometimes need a little push to get started.

Chapter 24:
Getting The Best Weight Loss Tips

Well, we all want to look fit and sexy all the time. Hence, we strive hard just to get the body that we want. However, with the lifestyle and eating habits that we were brought up with, it is almost impossible to stay slim and so easy to gain weight.

What with all the calories that we take in everyday, with all the junk and fast foods that we eat as well as the caffeinated beverages that we drink.

And in our desperation to trim down excess fats, we are always seeking for weight loss tips and different means to loss weight.

There are lots of tips available for you when it comes to losing weight. Books and magazines about weight loss as well as other essential things in losing weight are now within your reach.

Visit your favorite bookstores and magazine shops and you"ll surely find them.

Do-It-Yourself Weight Loss Tips

As there are a lot of tips on how to trim down excess fats and shed extra pounds that have been published, you can now easily find a set of procedures fitted for you and you lifestyle.

However, the best procedures to losing extra pounds are those which you can do even when you"re all by yourself; those which don't require you to go and consult a clinic or a weight loss expert.

Here are some weight loss tips that you can do yourself;

• Trim down your calories consumption

We need calories for our day to day activities, but we need to trim down unnecessary percentage of calories. Mostly, you may need to avoid soft drinks and alcoholic drinks. Gourmet coffee also contains too much calories and you may want to reduce consumption of this or totally avoid intake.

• Exercise is still a best way to shed extra pounds

Yes, this is still among the best practices that you can do at home to trim down extra pounds. You can start off by moving more often. Like instead of driving to a nearby supermarket, you can walk. Avoid riding if it is just a walking distance. You can also walk your dog every morning. Cleaning the house also makes your body move more often. You see, you don't need trainers and equipments just to exercise.

• Feast on 5 small meals everyday

Instead of eating 3 heavy meals, you can eat several small meals throughout the day. This way, you can divide your daily calorie intake without having to undergo fasting or skipping meals.

• Always eat breakfast

It is not a good idea to skip on breakfast just to lose weight. You will only tend to eat more later in the day.

• Water therapy

Water may not be considered as something which can burn fat, but drinking the right amount of water everyday can help with bodily functions such as proper digestion. It also makes you feel full so you won't feel like eating and eating.

If you haven't noticed, the tips above mostly involved self discipline. This is because discipline is the fundamental of all the weight loss procedures out there.

You have to know your limitations if you are serious about trimming down those unwanted fats. No weight loss tips are as effective as they promise if you, as the person who wants to lose weight, won't have even a bit of self discipline.

Chapter 25:
Healthy Ways To Lose Weight

You would be surprised at the number of strange and dangerous things that are sold as health products nowadays. People looking for a healthy way to lose weight will be bombarded by all kinds of foreign concoctions, supposed secrets of oriental doctors, that claim to allow them to lose weight the healthy way.

In reality however, you have no way of knowing what is really in these products. The healthiest way to lose weight is simply to start a healthy lifestyle.

I know all this from experience. You see, I have had a fluctuating weight problem for years and years. I get heavy from eating junk food or from failing to use good portion control and then lose all of that weight back very quickly.

I have used everything to lose weight quickly. I've even taken strange pills that make my heart race. They were advertised as a healthy way to lose weight. Let me tell you, these products are not healthy. There is a healthy way to lose weight, and it is very obvious. Exercise and keep a healthy diet.

A weight loss diet is not necessarily a healthy one. Many of the so-called healthy ways to lose weight actually put a great deal of strain on your body. Using some new fad such as the Atkins diet which requires you to eat massive amounts of fat and protein is not a healthy way to lose weight.

If your common sense is not enough to tell you this, you should look at the research. Many experts have linked the Atkins diet to liver shutdown. Weight loss should be good for you. It should not threaten your health.

If you have struggled with chronic weight problems all your life (as I have) and still have not found a healthy way to lose weight, it is time to get some support. You can do many things to find a healthy way to lose weight. You can join Weight Watchers, you can join a gym and get a personal trainer, or you can make a pact with some friends to encourage each other to eat right and exercise regularly.

Many of us overeat because we feel stressed out and disconnected. Just having a support group can be a healthy way to lose weight. It is always good for you to have friends who encourage you to do what is best for your health.

Chapter 26:
Natural Remedies For Losing Weight - Aloe

Normally when you think of aloe (which contains over 400 different species), you think of it being used for wound healing and things like burns. Aloe is actually added to herbal weight loss products for the main reason that it cleans you right out. It induces a strong cathartic response, which is why they also say on the labels it is an internal cleanser. One of the 400 species is Aloe Vera, and it is purported to have medicinal properties. Many cosmetics companies use aloe in their products and market them as skin rejuvenators.

Aloe has been touted as a cure all for coughs, wounds, ulcers and gastritis as well as arthritis and immune system deficiencies when taken internally. Apparently the only actual substantiated internal use is as a laxative.

Research on Aloe as a weight loss agent seems to consistently indicate it has no effect on weight loss despite its inclusion in over-the-counter natural remedies for losing weight. Many feel its inclusion is misleading to consumers.

An internal cleanser, when not spelled out that it promotes strong bowel movements, can mean many things, including it cleans up your system and rids you of fats. Certainly it may lead to some minimal weight loss, due to the time spent recycling the product. However, the real weight loss would come with a change in your diet and exercise program.

Aloe evidently also has some rather disturbing side effects - abdominal cramping, diarrhea, electrolyte disturbances, and decreases in potassium. It is also recommended you do not take aloe in combination with medications such as digoxin or diuretics.

The choice is yours and you can decide whether or not you want to try Aloe after you have read all you can about it. Most definitely it is being promoted as being effective in weight loss and not just because it causes diarrhea. It is said to reduce and stabilize body mass index by stimulating the metabolic rate in liver cells causing us to burn more energy. The other point about Aloe is that is has a high collagen protein content. Meaning, using aloe vera as a supplement in your diet would increase protein intake. The body spends more time trying to digest proteins and spends more energy doing that - thus it burns fat. It's baffling, but as always, talk to your Doctor.

Chapter 27:
Natural Weight Loss Remedies - Ayurveda

Being overweight or even morbidly obese seems to be quite a common problem worldwide. Ayurveda, perhaps more a methodology, is considered a good natural way to lose weight. It breaks human bodies into two categories - the very thin and the very fat. Fat bodies struggle with more diseases like high blood pressure, diabetes, arthritis, and gall bladder problems.

The main philosophy behind Ayurveda is the belief that being over-weight is due mainly to overeating, irregular eating habits and not properly balancing meals.

To that end, they highly recommend natural weight loss home remedies - a diet you can easily follow at home. Please remember, even this approach recommends exercising regularly. Ayurveda promotes using more fruits and green veggies, avoid too much salt, and avoid fat rich dairy products, meat and non-vegetarian foods.

Use dry ginger, cinnamon, and black pepper (fat burners). Avoid rice and potatoes, but go with a wheat based cereal.

Eat bitter gourd, and take honey as it mobilizes fat deposits (10 gms daily in hot water with 1 tsp of lemon juice). Try a lime/honey fast to keep energy levels up. Juice of half a lime, 1 tsp fresh honey in lukewarm water at regular intervals.

Cabbage is touted for inhibiting the conversion of sugar and other carbs into fat. Eat raw or cooked. And, make your portions smaller. Supplements are also suggested like Ezi Slim, Medohar Vidangadi Lauh, Punarnavadi Guggul and Neemguard.

Evidently Neemguard (Neem, Giloy and Triphala)is considered safe for increasing the metabolism to reduce your weight and the Indian herb guggulu (a gum resin obtained from the plant of Balsamo-dendron mukul) is the drug of choice for treating obesity.

Many of the herbs used in other countries, while likely effective, may be of questionable use to you if you are not sure just what they are, and what they do. Although the Ayurveda supplements are herbal and natural, you might want to check with your Doctor before embarking on a weight loss program like this.

Chapter 28:

Natural Remedies For Losing Weight - Bitter Orange

It seems that Bitter Orange(Citrus aurantium aka sour orange, bigarade orange and Seville orange) is the "other" ephedra, and as such has similar side effects. Natural remedies for losing weight that have Bitter Orange in them are marketed as Ephedra Free when in reality their chemical make up is almost a mirror image of the ephedrine in Ephedra. This is just one reason why you need to be carefully reading labels and researching ingredients on any product you are considering for your weight loss journey.

Bitter Orange contains synephrine and octopamine, chemicals that may cause high blood pressure, and heart disturbances. This herbal can also inhibit the metabolism of many drugs meaning it would increase the amount of the drug in your body and the risk of adverse side effects. You have to stop and ask yourself if risking your health if worth it under these circumstances when you can lose weight by merely changing your diet and exercising.

Bitter orange as well as bitter orange peel is not recommended for use in isolation - for instance, in traditional

Chinese medicine, it is prescribed in support with other herbs by experienced herbalists. The flower of the bitter orange is used for poor appetite, chest and stomach pain, and vomiting. Homeopathic practitioners use the peel and flower for headaches and pain. Only the peel has proven medicinal value, mainly for digestive problems. It does appear that the several compounds in Bitter Orange will stimulate metabolic rates, but no clinical trials have actually proven this. It may be that Bitter Orange is effect when combined with St. John's Wort and Caffeine.

However, this means three stimulants all at once. Even in the best of circumstances, taking three known stimulants in one preparation is not a good idea. Most natural remedies for losing weight that use Bitter Orange made from concentrated extract of the peel contain anywhere from 1 to 6 per cent synephine. Unfortunately, this could vary up to amounts of about 30 per cent or more depending or what part of the plant was used and how it was processed.

Bottom line? Use extreme caution when taking any herbal remedies that contain so many stimulants. Always ask your Doctor or an experienced herbalist about these preparations before taking them.

Chapter 29:
Natural Remedies For Losing Weight
- Cascara

Cascara Sagrada (also called Sacred Bark, Bitter Bark, Chittem bark , California Buckthorn and Rhamnus purshiana) is a common ingredient found in natural remedies for losing weight. A strong stimulant laxative, it needs to be used with a great deal of care because it can leech potassium and sodium from your body. Of interest, the bark of the tree is removed, cut into small pieces, and dried for one year before being used medicinally.

Spanish priests in California named the tree Cascara is harvested from. It's name origins may either be from the medicinal properties of the bark or from its resemblance to wood used for the ark of the covenant.

Most Doctors will advice you that Cascara should be taken consecutively for no longer than eight to ten days, so you need to very carefully read labels when considering a natural remedy for losing weight that contains cascara.

If pregnant or nursing, you must also use this with extreme caution.

It seems the main raison d'etre of this herbal product is to promote bowel movements, so how does it figure in today's natural remedies for losing weight? Many of the products being marketed that have Cascara in them are packaged with other products to supposedly give you a lean look, help you become a fat burning furnace and so forth. This is precisely this thing you need to be careful of when you read labels.

If you find yourself reading a label that has Cascara, psyllium husks and Senna(all bowel movement enhancers), and Valerian (for sleeplessness) and an appetite suppress-ant, and a whole list of other ingredients, head for your Pharmacist to translate for you. It may be that using a product like this helps you lose weight because you are continually expelling what you do eat with the aid of bowel stimulators.

Not a healthy way to lose weight. While Senna, Cascara, and Aloe are authorized for oral use as laxatives, they are also way too often promoted for detoxifying or cleansing regimens. There are serious risks with the chronic use of laxatives or combining multiple laxatives together. These can include the risk of electrolyte disturbances affecting the heart, as well as functional bowel problems. Use cau-tion when investigating herbal substances for weight loss.

Chapter 30:
Natural Remedies For Losing Weight
- Chromium

Chromium, also referred to as Chromium Picolinate (a combination of chromium and picolinic acid), is a supposedly a miracle mineral that's just the bee's knees when it comes too natural remedies for losing weight.

It is supposed to promote weight loss, enhance your moods, boost energy, and even let you live a longer life.

This is actually a very popular weight loss aid and is supposed to melt fat, reduce appetite and kick up your metabolism. Sounds pretty good doesn't it? Who wouldn't want all those benefits in today's "obsessed with losing weight" culture. Interestingly enough, Chromium Picolinate is being promoted as a safe alternative to taking steroids.

The claim is it increases strength and lean muscle mass. Obviously the manufacturers have been doing a good job of marketing this product as you will readily find it in hundreds of locations - health food stores, drugstores and even on the Internet.

How is this supposed to work? Chromium Picolinate works by stimulating the activity of insulin, significantly assisting the body's breakdown of glucose and fat. Some dieters claim the improved insulin efficiency causes an increase in seratonin, which reduces appetite. Others say chromium can prevent excess fat from forming. Whatever the actual truth of the matter is, it may remain a mystery for some time yet.

The bottom line is it may work for some people, and not others. It may suppress appetite or not. If it makes you feel better about your weight loss efforts, then go for it. You will still need a program though that will help you succeed in keeping the fat off.

There are so many differing opinions on this product that it's best to take some time and do your own research. Many swear by its ability to suppress appetite and thus promote weight loss. Others don't believe it can do what it claims to be able to deliver. The only person who can decide is you.

Talk to people you know, read all you can get your hands on, and talk to your medical professional. Then, when you have enough information to make an informed choice, do what feels right for you.

Chapter 31:
Natural Remedies For Losing Weight
- Chitosan

This natural remedy for losing weight has a fascinating history and a ton of really useful things it is used for, not the least of which is supposedly being at fat attractant. One thing to note if you are considering trying this natural remedy for weight loss - if you have shellfish allergies do not take this product.

Chitosan is made from something called chitin - a starch found in shrimp, crab and other shellfish skeletons. It's most common uses are: As a plant growth enhancer, and defender against fungal infections. As a filtration component in water processing engineering that binds sediment and removes it. It also removes phosphorus, heavy minerals, and oils from water. As a clarifying agent for wine, mead and beer that removes yeast cells, fruit particles etc As a blood clotter, used in bandages. Hypoallergenic with natural anti-bacterial properties. But, what about weight loss? Where does Chitosan fit into losing weight. Here's where the fat attractent theory comes into play. It's frequently sold health food stores and billed as a substance that attracts fat from the digestive system and expels it from the body.

This in theory means a dieter could lose weight without eating less. Unfortunately, it appears to be just that, a theory. Research has shown unmodified Chitosan would possibly remove about 30 calories a day from a person's diet. Modified, this product boasts claims (mostly unsubstantiated) of absorbing from three to six times its weight in fat and oil. Evidently initial trials with the product to test its effectiveness as a weight loss remedy were conducted on animals, not humans.

So most of the speculation about what this product can or can not do is moot and just that, speculation. It seems most weight loss professionals agree that Chitosan doesn't do the job when it comes to weight loss. And what recent trials there have been only show no more weight loss than a person who took placebo sugar pills.

Chitosan (KITE-o-san). This dietary supplement is made from chitin, a starch found in the skeleton of shrimp, crab, and other shellfish. Chitosan cannot be digested; therefore it passes through your intestinal tract unabsorbed without adding any calories. The chemical nature of Chitosan makes it bind with fatty foods, removing some of the fat from your body as it passes through rather than allowing it to be absorbed. Several studies, however, found no more weight loss from Chitosan than from a placebo (sugar pill).

Chapter 34:
Natural Remedies For Losing Weight - Dandelion

The lowly Dandelion, the usual grass destroying culprit in our yards that gets cut on a regular basis with the lawn-mower, is known by a variety of names such as lion's tooth, fairy clock, priest's crown, swine's snout, blowball, milk gowan, and wild endive.   In addition to medicinal uses, dandelion can be used as a food and beverage. Leaves can be used raw in salads and sandwiches, or for tea. Roots can make a coffee substitute and the flowers can be used for wine and schnapps.

In Europe, the dandelion was used to treat fevers, boils, diarrhea, fluid retention, heartburn, and various skin problems. The Chinese used dandelion to treat breast cancer, inflammation, lack of milk flow, liver diseases, and digestive problems.

As far as weight loss is concerned, the dandelion is considered to be a natural diuretic. It may produce significant weight loss by decreasing body water. However, it can cause allergic reactions and heartburn.

Weight control is definitely an obsession worldwide. In the US alone, two-thirds of the adult population is overweight and one third is classified as obese. It is any wonder that the natural herbal weight loss industry now offers more than 50 supplements and 125 proprietary products for weight loss. The question is have they been thoroughly tested to see if they live up to their claims.

Dandelion has been around for a long time, and thus has a history to support its claims. Those who support the use of dandelion in weight loss claim it may flush out the kidneys, boost metabolism, and cut your craving for sweets. How? Eating the leaves raw in a salad, or making tea and drinking it three times a day.

These may trim pounds in short order thanks to the diuretic effect, but continued use can cause dehydration and electrolyte abnormalities. You need to read all you can about any weight loss products before you try them.

For safe weight loss, your best bet would be to use the tried and true methods of changing your eating habits and exercising more.

Chapter 35:
Natural Remedies For Losing Weight
- Dexatrim

Many will remember the almost famous Dexatrim weight loss capsules. They've been around in so many different formulations it is almost difficult to keep up with them. They've so far been through three reincarnations, none of which seems to be all that effective in terms of being able to lose weight.

Formulation number one contained phenylpropanolamine and was banned in 2001 because of its links to strokes. Formulation number two came out awhile later, and its main ingredient was ephedra also recalled in 2002 because it was cited as causing strokes, heart attacks and death. The manufactruing company is now on incarnation number three and the main ingredient this time is Bitter Orange Peel extract. - now known as the other Ephedra of the weight loss industry.

The Bitter Orange is combined with a few other proprietary ingredients - which usually means they've just selected other herbals to combine and boost the main ingredient - such as Yohimbe Bark (side effects like bitter orange, high blood pressure, palpitations, headache), Siberian Ginseng (safe), Licorice root (high doses cause high blood pressure), and so on. If you have been counting, there are at least three ingredients in this that can cause high blood pressure. Can you imagine the effect it may possibly have on you?

Various formulations of Dexatrim have various ingredients in each, all of which would need to be checked and cross referenced. For instance, in one of their blends, the main ingredient is green tea extract - the only herbal ingredient that has been shown to suppress appetite without side effects.

But you certainly do not need to be buying a formulation with green tea extract and several other dubious weight loss products when you can buy a whole box of tea bags for about three dollars.

Even though the company that makes Dexatrim (Chettem) has reinvented its weight loss products three times, it still isn't something that is considered to be safe or effective for long term weight loss results. The only long term effective weight loss program is eating less and exercising more.

Chapter 36:
Natural Remedies For Losing Weight
- Ephedra

Most natural remedies, or over-the-counter (OTC) herbal medicines for weight loss have appetite suppressants in them. That only makes sense, as you want to stop eating as much. The appetite killers trick your body into thinking it's not really hungry. Short-term use isn't bad. Long-term use can lead to serious problems. Despite taking any of these natural remedies for losing weight, you still need to make major changes in your diet and exercise program.

One of the more commonly used OTC natural weight loss remedies is Ephedra, aka Ma-Huang harvested from the Ephedra sinica plant. Interestingly enough, this plant has been used in traditional Chinese medicine for over 5,000 years for asthma, hay fever and the common cold. Native Americans and Mormon pioneers drank Mormon Tea, brewed from Ephedra.

In 2004, it was banned after it came under fire for danger-ous side effects and was cited as the culprit in several deaths. As of February 2007, the sale of dietary supple-ments containing ephedra is illegal in the USA. If you think this would work for you in your weight loss program, then the best thing to do is talk to your Doctor. It's better to be fully informed than to get a nasty surprise.

Ma Huang or Ephedra has been commonly found in herbal dietary supplements for years. It also happens to be used in the manufacture of methamphetamine (speed).

Its greatest claim to fame was that it suppressed the appetite so you would not eat as much - which would mean you'd lose weight, but it has not been clinically proven to be effective in weight loss. Which is also interesting,
because Ephedra is a stimulant and thermogenic.

The brain is stimulated, heart rate increased, blood pressure increased and bronchial tubes expand. The thermogenic properties cause an increase in metabolism, which will usually start to burn off body fat. While this all sounds good, the down side to this natural remedy for losing weight is that it could literally kill you.

Either because of the side effects, or because of a drug interaction with something else you may be taking. Seriously consider if this is really something you want to try.

Chapter 37:
Natural Remedies For Losing Weight - Garcinia (hydroxycitric Acid - Hca)

Garcinia Cambogia hails from India and Southeast Asia and is a pumpkin shaped fruit with a chemical structure similar to citric acid. Also called Malabar Tamarind, you will find this as a condiment in curry dishes.

HCA apparently does reduce appetites and promotes weight loss in animals, as proven by several studies. However, when humans were studied, it was found HCA did not burn excess calories. In fact, it was labeled as no better than a sugar pill.

Many claims on diet and weight loss remedy packages insist there are no side effects for HCA. No one seems to be sure whether there is or isn't which doesn't bode well for HCA as a natural remedy for losing weight.

Bottom line? It's really unclear whether or not HCA offers weight loss benefits or not. The best that can be said about it is that it likely won't hurt you, although no real studies have been done addressing whether or not it's safe to take long term, or take at all.

One double blind study found of 60 overweight people who used 440 mg of HCA 3 times a day showed weight loss.

Yet another study (also double blind) of 135 overweight individuals who got either 500 mg of HCA or a placebo 3 times a day bombed out - showed no effects re: weight loss. The best available data today shows this product is not effective for weight loss.

You will definitely have to think long and hard about this particular product, even if you choose to use it in combination with another weight loss remedy.

If you are gong to be spending money to buy products with dubious track records, then you are likely getting what you paid for.

Try and thoroughly research HCA or any other natural remedy for losing weight to find out the pros and the cons before you take a leap of faith into something that might not work.

Chapter 38: Natural Remedies For Losing Weight - Guar Gum

So many people these days want a magic bullet to lose weight, actually fervently pray for such a thing. Unfortunately, there really is NO magic bullet for weight loss, other than good old hard work to make it happen.

No matter what else you choose to do, you still need to change your eating habits, and increase your exercise. Why are these natural remedies for losing weight so popular?

There are numerous reasons why the natural weight loss industry does a booming business every year. Over weight and obese people want something they can lose weight with immediately.

It's easier that doing the grunt work. They have decided they don't want to be fat any longer and want instant results.

They may have tried other weight loss avenues and given up. Herbal remedies are easy to obtain without a prescription.

They appeal to people because of the outrageous claims made about weight loss. People think natural can't hurt you and that natural means safe - and it doesn't.

Hundreds of weight loss products have soluble fiber in them, meaning in theory, the fiber will absorb water in your gut, decreasing your appetite, making you feel full and not eat as much.

Guar gum (from the cluster bean Cyamopsis tetragonolobus) is one of these fibers used as a natural remedy for losing weight.

The guar seeds are dehusked, milled and screened to obtain the guar gum. Normally, you would find this thickening agent in foods, dairy products, sauces and ice cream. Used in food it is quite easy for the body to assimilate it. Used in diet concoctions, that is another kettle of fish.

Since it is capable of swelling up to 10 to 20 times in the stomach when taken with fluids, it is supposed to make you feel full, cut your appetite, making you eat less, and thus losing weight.

Unfortunately, there have been many instances of esophageal blockages with this product. Like Glocomannan, Guar gum has also led to gastrointestinal obstructions.

Research indicates that this product was banned in the US in over-the-counter natural remedies for losing weight in the late 1980s. In addition, Guar gum was also proved ineffective in losing weight.

However, with the exploding weight loss market, always be sure to read labels before you buy something. You will find that many things are called by other names and if you do not know what they are, you could buy something that will either by a waste of your money, or cause you more problems than you ever wanted.

Chapter 39:
Natural Remedies For Losing Weight
- Herbal Diuretics

Hundreds upon hundreds of people have at one time or another struggled to lose weight. It's a really important issue for many since society places such value on being thin. Do you realize that over 300,000 people a month search the Internet using the term weight loss?

Billions of dollars have been spent on weight loss and the weight loss industry is making money hand over fist. Oddly enough, even though there are all these natural remedies for losing weight on the market, obesity is on the rise. People and children are fatter than ever.

The natural weight loss remedies gear themselves to people just like this - praying on their dreams to be thinner, their frustration at not being able to lose and their confusion over what will or will not work for them.

If you have ever read any of the labels for natural weight loss products, you'll likely realize more than half the ingredients have names you likely do not recognize.

And most definitely you will not know how they interact with one another, and with any drugs you may be taking. That's the bad news. The good news is you can lose weight, but you need to do it the old fashioned way change your diet and get exercise. There is simply no way around that. Back to reading labels, and trying to figure out what is in the product you are looking at. Many of the over-the-counter weight loss products have a variety of herbal diuretics in them, and most of them are derived from caffeine (which is a stimulant).

Some of them have juniper seeds (can cause renal failure), equistine (a neurotoxin - can cause brain damage), horse tail or shave grass (convulsions/hyperactivity). There is also dandelion, hawthorn and green tea.

By themselves, herbal diuretics don't provide enough water shedding to give you an effective water weight loss. And while not considered to be toxic (on their own) when mixed with a variety of other compounds they can have serious interactions with drugs you may be taking already to achieve weight loss (like Lasix). In addition if you are on lithium or digoxin herbal diuretics have a history of interacting with these medications. Herbal diuretics trick you into thinking you are getting thinner. You're not. You are merely losing water weight. If you take these kinds of products too long, the loss of water will leach sodium and potassium from your body. The best method to achieve the same effect is drink lots of purified water.

Chapter 40:
Natural Remedies For Losing Weight
- 5-hydroxytryptophan (5-htp)

Another natural remedy for losing weight that has raised a few eyebrows is a substance called 5-hydroxytryptophan (5-HTP). In fact, its been called into question for its safety record. 5-HTP actually replaced tryptophan supplements banned due to its link to a rare and potentially deadly blood disorder. Also, there has been a difference of opinion on whether or not it is actually a viable substance for achieving weight loss. Now, having said that, 5-HTP is found in some over-the-counter natural remedies for losing weight.

5-HTP is used to make serotonin for normal nerve and brain function. Lack of it affects sleep, emotional moods, pain control, inflammation, intestinal peristalsis (acts as a stimulant), and other body functions. It's found in the cells of the brain(acts as a neurotransmitter speeding nerve impulses between synapses) and intestine and in platelets in our blood. When walls of blood vessels are damaged, serotonin is released from platelets to constrict the vessel and prevent hemorrhage.

The human body doesn't make a lot of this. 5-HTP is derived from the seeds of a West African plant called Griffonia simplicifoli. Dieters who use this product claim it helps suppress appetite, and helps promote weight loss.

Initial research says 5-HTP is noted for its ability to reduce appetite by stimulating serotonin production in the brain. Clinical trials have appetite reduction and weight loss (averaging 11 pounds in 12 weeks) with 600 to 900 mg daily. Trials using 5-HTP did show that some people taking large amounts of 5-HTP had nausea, headaches, sleepiness, muscle pain, or anxiety.

With this natural remedy for losing weight, and others as well, you must change your eating habits and increase exercise. It will not work all that well just on its own.

In addition, if you happen to be pregnant or nursing, check with a Doctor, as there is no research in this area to indicate whether it is safe to take this substance under these circumstances.

Try not to get taken in with the common belief that if it is natural, it won't hurt you. Nothing could be further from the truth. Get as much information as you can before you decide to try anything.

Chapter 41:
Natural Remedies For Losing Weight
- Leptoprin

The bottom line with natural remedies for losing weight is that if you stop taking them, the weight comes back. You have not learned anything about how to properly lose weight and maintain your loss. You have tricked your body into perhaps losing some fat and likely some water - but have not addressed the underlying causes as to why you may be overweight in the first place. If there actually were a diet pill that worked for the long term you can bet major drug companies would be selling them. They aren't!

Leptoprin (Anorex) has Calcium Phosphate, Commiphora mukul extract, Garcinia cambogia (HCA 125mg), L-Tyrosine, Acetylsalicyclic acid - 162.5mg, Dipotassium phosphate, Sodium phosphate, Disodium phosphate, Phosphatidyl choline, Scutellaria (root), Bupleurum (root), Epimedium (herb). You might be asking, as you should, why a diet product would have aspirin in it (something people on Coumadin dare not take).

Leptoprin is something called a Stack. The ECA (ephedra, caffeine and aspirin) stack is supposedly a thermogenic product - meaning it supposedly melts your fat away by boosting your metabolism. And while it may boost your metabolism, it is more than likely to give you a bad case of the jitters with two stimulants tag teamed together. It's like taking speed, as there is only a minimal difference between methamphetamine and ephedrine/ephedra.

The side effects for a product like this are many - irregular or accelerated heart beat, insomnia, elevated blood pressure, seizures etc. And yet these products are labeled all natural. This is misleading as people then think they are also harmless.

Again, as with any natural remedies, read the labels, search for the names of the list ingredients on the Internet, check for drug interactions, talk to your Doctor and/or your Pharmacist.

If you're considering taking something like this, it is better to be well informed, and have your Doctor know what you are doing. In the long run, you would best be served by a visit to your local Weight Watchers group and find out how they can help you with a truly natural weight loss program.

Chapter 42:
Natural Remedies For Losing Weight
- Pyruvate

It seems we all have Pyruvate present in our bodies, as it is formed during the digestion of carbohydrates and proteins. The claims for this natural remedy for losing weight are that it reduces fat, prevents the fat loss yo-yo effect, reduces cholesterol and increases endurance.
All very beneficial things, if they actually come to pass.

And now down to business, does this work or doesn't it? Again, you would definitely need to do your own research as there seems to be at least three difference answers to that question - yes, no and maybe in some cases.

Some say it works but only at high dosages (22 - 28 grams daily when the recommended dose is 500 micrograms to 1 gram). Some studies show that 23 per cent of the people who participated actually lost weight as opposed to some claims of a 48 per cent weight loss (roughly 2 to 3 pounds, not significant).

Now, on the other hand, another body of research says pyruvate does affect weight loss by burning fat and boosts energy. And this, good for high-end athletes and body builders, it kicks up the transport of glucose and protein into muscle cells and boosts exercise performance levels. Translation: helps them get toned and have more energy.

Once again, the jury is out on whether Pyruvate is truly effective or not. One thing you can take to the bank is that Pyruvate can be found in red apples, cheese and red wine. That's not to say go out and stuff yourself with any or all of these foods. But it does indicate that small amounts may be just fine, where larger amounts may be problematic.

In the final analysis, more study is needed to determine if Pyruvate's claims of decreasing appetite and helping you lose weight are actually valid. What is certain, is this product is highly touted as a natural remedy for losing weight. The decision is up to you. Weigh all the options with care.

Chapter 43:
Natural Remedies For Losing Weight
- St. John's Wort

There's definitely a large number of natural remedies for losing weight on the market, the question really becomes how effective are they and how safe are they.
The answers to both of those questions would need to be researched carefully before you made any decisions. One thing to also remember, if you happen to be morbidly obese, many of these natural remedies for losing weight are likely not for you. As with any weight loss venture, you need to make sure you talk to your Doctor before you start any program.

One rather controversial herbal product that has a history of actually being used as an anti-depressant, seems to also be another contender in the weight loss arena. St. John's Wort, also called Hypericum, Klamath Weed, or Goat Weed, has been used for centuries to treat nerve pain, mental disorders, malaria, insect bites, wounds and burns. Amazingly, there are over 370 species of the genus Hypericum worldwide. It was also used by Native American as an anti-inflammatory, antiseptic and astringent.

In the twentieth century St. John's Wort (named for its traditional flowering and harvesting on St. John's day, June 24th) has more commonly been used to treat depression, anxiety, and/or sleep disorders. The part of the plant used to make preparations is the top of the little yellow flower and is usually used to makes teas and tablets.

How does St John's Wort help you lose weight? That's the funny part - it does and it doesn't. It seems the herbal remedy itself does not help you lose weight. However, how it makes you feel by improving how you feel about yourself, does cause you to lose weight. Being in a better frame of mind may cause people to eat less. Bottom line is any change in your eating habits after taking St. John's Wort will have more to do with any psychological improvements and not the herbal remedy.

Here's the most interesting thing though, there are natural remedies for losing weight on the market that feature St. John's Wort as the main active ingredient. The way it's presented implies St. John's Wort is the key proponent to your anticipated weight loss. It isn't, and this is a misrepresentation. So once again, do your research before you start taking any natural remedies for losing weight. Also, pay attention to any side-effects that may result from the herbal remedy you are considering.

Chapter 44:
Natural Remedies For Losing Weight
- The Brain/mind

This might seem like an usual idea, losing weight using the brain/mind - but if you stop to think about it - it makes perfect sense. Where do all your thoughts come from? You decision making abilities? Your fears, joys, etc? The brain/mind. It's far more powerful than many give it credit for and sadly underestimated as well.

Let's think about this idea a bit more - the brain as a natural remedy for losing weight. Not only is it immediately at your disposal, it is free. It's always available and can perform amazing feats when given the chance. You've heard and read about the power of positive thinking, about affirmations and meditation. They work, so why wouldn't being positive about your weight loss journey?

How difficult would it be to re-tool thinking patterns about food, diets, lifestyle changes and exercising? It might take quite a long time, but if the motivation is there, and the will and drive to succeed, it would make a winning combination. Granted there are exceptions to every rule, and there no doubt would be people who are genetically disposed to weight gain, those who have medical reasons they cannot lose weight, and still others who just don't want to lose weight for their own reasons.

In the final analysis, using your mind/brain connection in combination with a change in eating habits, increased exercise, smaller portions, and weight loss support groups certainly won't hurt you. In fact, it may teach you about a whole other side to how powerful your mind/brain can really be. It won't give you side effects either.

That is the key to the weight loss industry, it prays on our mind and our fears about being overweight. It sends subtle negative messages that tell you to rely on drugs for a solution you really have control over. The hundreds of weight loss remedies mostly suggest you cannot lose weight without this herb or that fat burner.

A few will mention in small print that you should change your lifestyle in addition to using their products, but let's face it, how many people actually take the time to read the small print. With a little planning, a powerful urge to succeed in losing weight, a positive mind/brain approach to the changes you need to make and support and hard work - you WILL make it, there is no doubt about it.

Chapter 45:
Dangers Of Using Laxatives For Weight Loss

One popular weight loss supplement available in the market today takes the form of tea. Stores all over sell slimming tea, dieter's tea and others but all of them are actually the same. They may appear to be effective, but what is not seen may actually harm you.

One of the effects of drinking dieter's tea is frequent bowel movement. This gives people the feeling of body cleansing. These people may get toxins out of their body but it isn't exactly the only thing that slimming tea actually does to the body.

Slimming tea contains herbs which are natural laxatives. These include aloe, senna, rhubarb root, cascara, buck-thorn and castor oil. These are products which are derived from plants and are used since the ancient times because of their potency in treating constipation and to inducing bowel movement.

Cascara, castor oil and senna are substances which are recognized as laxatives available over the counter and are also regulated as drugs. Scientific studies show that diarrhea induced by laxatives does not absorb significant amounts of calories taken in the body.

The reason for this is that laxatives do not act on the small intestines where most of the calories are absorbed. Instead, they work on the large intestines. If taken in large amounts for prolonged periods, it can affect fat absorption of the body.

This may lead to greasy diarrhea and loss of weight. Abuse of laxatives is common practice among people who suffer from bulimia and anorexia nervosa.

While weight loss can be guaranteed by overdosing on laxatives, it may also cause permanent damage to the gastrointestinal tract and the weakening and softening of the bones, a condition known as osteomalacia.

Drinkers of slimming teas may actually patronize the product because they are less expensive and taste better than other laxatives sold in the market.

Other people, such as those with eating disorders like bulimia and anorexia nervosa drink dieter's tea because they work fast and produce watery stool and having loose consistency.

Women may even be more susceptible to the effects of slimming teas. Although they are not known to interfere directly with the woman's menstrual cycle and fertility, they should watch out if drinking them causes them to rapidly shed off weight.

It is also not safe for pregnant women to be taking in laxatives of any kind. Wise and responsible herbalists also discourage the use of senna and other herbal products with laxative properties for pregnant women and women who are trying to conceive.

One should be wary about these findings because the labeling of slimming teas in the market today can be absolutely misleading. For instance, they commonly refer to the laxative qualities as "natural bowel cleansing properties" and not specifically use the word "laxative".Some even use the term "low-calorie" on their labeling.

These products in fact, contain essentially no calories nor nutrients whatsoever; unless of course, if they are sweetened.

Adverse effects of misusing laxatives in the form of slimming tea generally occur when taken in more than or longer than recommended.

These include nausea, stomach cramps, vomiting, diarrhea, fainting, rectal bleeding,electrolyte disorder and dehydration as well as injury and worse, death.

It was also reported that excess use of stimulant laxatives cause severe constipation and pain for long periods (as much as for decades) due to the colon losing its function. It eventually led to surgery removing the colon altogether.

Chapter 46:
Natural Remedies For Losing Weight - Yerba Mate

Yerba Mate (Ilex paraguariensis) belongs to the holly family and is prepared by steeping dry leaves and twigs in hot water (the infusion is called Mate). Only slightly less potent than coffee, it appears to be easier on the stomach. Yerba Mate has a strong vegetable, herbal, and grassy flavor much like some varieties of green tea. Over the past few years, extracts of Yerba Mate have shown upin natural remedies for losing weight. Why? Because it contains over 250 natural compounds such as caffeine, theophylline and theobromine.

These compounds stimulate the central nervous system, and are diuretics, causing the body to shed water. Caffeine, theophylline and theobromine suppress appetite, and boost metabolism.

The question is if Yerba Mate contains these ingredients and they are then combined with other variations of stimulants, diuretics, fat burners and goodness knows what else, what kind of side effects are potentially lurking in the wings?

Yerba Mate proponents insist this is one of those wonder herbals that can actually achieve your weight loss and leaner physique goals without having to do too much about exercise or changing how you eat.

They say Yerba mate suppresses appetite, increases caloric burn rate, and increases urination, thereby reducing overall body water weight. Note they say overall body WATER weight. While losing water does mean you weigh less, it doesn't address the primary problem of over eating, not eating properly and not exercising.

At best, it would seem this product may be more of a quick fix than a real weight loss product. Always check with a doctor about your weight loss goals and how you are going to achieve them.

If you plan on using an herbal product like this, then make sure your Doctor knows what other medications you are taking in addition. It is better to be safe, and to do your homework, rather than just plunge into something you aren't really sure about.

Chapter 47:
Ardyss Body Magic Garment

Finally there are body shaping garments that really work. The Ardyss Body Magic will instantly reduce your dress size, help improve your posture and strip the fat bulges off your figure. Ardyss Body Magic support combines fashion, orthopedics and technology to produce a remarkable change in your figure.

You can reduce your figure by two or three sizes instantly with this carefully designed undergarment, which will give your waist renewed definition, assist in slimming your thighs, and provide lift to the breasts – all without difficult, painful and expensive surgery.

In addition, Ardyss Body Magic garments were designed with the input of an orthopedic surgeon and clothing design professionals to support the lower back and help to straighten your posture. They apply even, consistent, comfortable pressure on where it can do the most good.

- Your abdomen will be flattened; contributing tone to those muscles and helping your abdominal organs function more efficiently.

- Buttocks are reshaped when Ardyss Body Magic design helps to round and/or reduce them.

- You'll be wearing a compression garment that eliminates those fatty lumps and both smooths and moves fat to places where it belongs.

- The lumbar and abdominal support will have you standing taller, in a position that naturally strengthens the muscles you need for a youthful figure.

- Ardyss Body Magic garments are designed to lift and reshape breasts as nature made them.

This comfortable, feminine garment will provide you with instant results, getting you off to a quick start in your weight loss efforts. There are a number of designs for our reshaping undergarments, for both men and women.

Our doctors, engineers and fashion designers are continuing to refine this revolutionary fat reduction concept and apply it in a variety of high-tech, highly attractive clothing options.

But for women who need that kick-start for launching a body improvement program, nothing will work better than an Ardyss Body Magic sheath that instantly shapes you, slims you and gives you a reason to supplement these results, if you choose, with dieting and exercise.

Learn more about Ardyss garments at www.buybodymagic.com

www.ingramcontent.com/pod-product-compliance
Lightning Source LLC
Chambersburg PA
CBHW072132280526
45788CB00002B/609